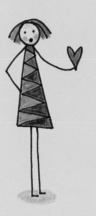

FOR MISS HAYNES

WITH LOVE AND

KINDNESS

Love

Méabh

xxx

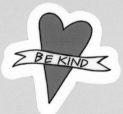

'What a timely and lovely book this is'
Russell Brand

'A hug in book form'
Emma Bunton

'Share the gift of kindness'
Holly Willoughby

'Let's make kindness a part of everything we do'
June Sarpong

'Kindness is free! So give it out! Give it to everyone'
Leigh Francis

'Kindness can be the most precious gift'
Melanie B

'The kindness you give always
comes back to you'
Ronnie Wood

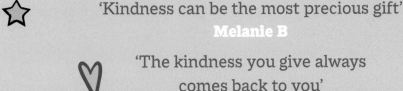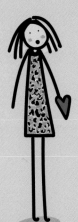

'Don't delay, be kind today'
Chris Evans

Rosie Nixon lives in London and is Editor-in-Chief of *HELLO!* magazine, where she has worked for over a decade. She is the author of three novels and *Be Kind* is her first non-fiction title. Rosie is a mother of two children and has worked in the women's magazine industry for over 20 years.

When she's not keeping on top of the latest royal and showbiz news, or dreaming up her latest creative writing project, Rosie is passionate about issues concerning women and children and their right to equality and is a proud ambassador of the charity SafeHands. She is a passionate believer in the power of kindness and loves talking about the subject.

Jakki Jones has worked with talent in the entertainment business for over 17 years. Outside of the day job she is a keen doodler and writer. When she's not penning her memoirs on motherhood, Jakki also likes to take part in live events and panels and is uber passionate about instilling kindness everywhere she goes.

Everyday inspiration featuring **Beverley Knight,**
Chris Evans, Dermot O'Leary, **Fearne Cotton,**
Holly Willoughby, June Sarpong,
Matt Haig, **Russell Brand**
and more...

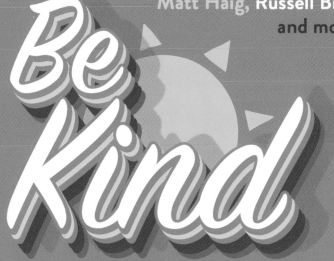

Be Kind

ROSIE NIXON, illustrated by **Jakki Jones**

An imprint of HarperCollinsPublishers Ltd.

HQ
An imprint of HarperCollins*Publishers* Ltd
1 London Bridge Street, London SE1 9GF

www.harpercollins.co.uk

HarperCollins*Publishers*
1st Floor, Watermarque Building, Ringsend Road, Dublin 4, Ireland

This edition 2021

1
First published in Great Britain by
HQ, an imprint of HarperCollinsPublishers Ltd 2021

ISBN: 978-0-00-847132-3

MIX
Paper from
responsible sources
FSC™ C007454

This book is produced from independently certified FSC™ paper to ensure responsible forest management.

For more information visit: www.harpercollins.co.uk/green

Designed by **Steve Wells**

Printed and bound by GPS Group, Slovenia

CONTENTS ♥

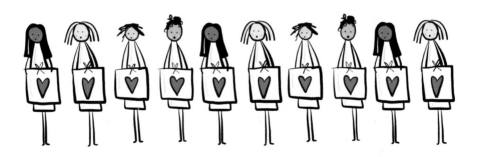

Dedications

This book is dedicated to our children.
Here's what they had to say about kindness:

'Kindness is being friendly and helpful.
Once you've done something kind it makes
you feel happy too, not just the person
you've been kind to.'
Heath, age 7

'Kindness is good manners.'
Rex, age 6

'Kindness is being gentle and really nice to
other people.'
Riley, age 5

Giggles
Marley, age 1

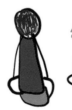

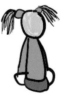
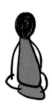

kindness

/ˈkʌɪn(d)nəs/

noun

1. the quality of being gentle, caring and helpful.

Collins English Dictionary

Introduction

Welcome to *Be Kind*.
A small book with a big heart
and an important message.
Kindness can change the world.
Yes, really! And it starts, today,
with you.

Kindness costs nothing; it isn't about grand gestures and it doesn't care who you are or where you are from. Kindness is within us all – but sometimes we need a gentle reminder, or a helping hand, to bring the power of kindness into our daily lives.
The smallest acts of kindness can be the most rewarding: a smile, a supportive message, making time to listen. Kindness builds self-confidence, it strengthens relationships, it has health benefits and it will always make your world a better place. You have a choice about how you will act in any

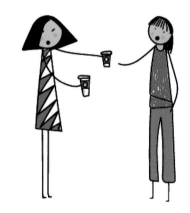

given situation and, I promise you, choosing the kind option will always be rewarding.

I started to think about kindness in depth during the course of my role as Editor-in-Chief of *HELLO!* magazine. At *HELLO!* we strongly believe in treating people with kindness and respect, whoever they are – from the famous personalities who grace our pages, to our readers, contributors and vast online audience – but when we launched our #hellotokindness campaign, I saw first-hand just how powerful collective kindness can be. We spearheaded this movement initially because we wanted to create a kinder, more supportive community on our social media channels; we wanted to make a stand to say that unkind or abusive commentary had no place in our world and to encourage users to 'think twice' before posting. The reaction to this was huge; it resonated strongly with our audience and large numbers joined our cause. Our platforms have become a kinder place as a result and a kind ethos continues to underpin everything we do.

Being guided by kindness has made my job more rewarding than I could possibly have imagined. It has enhanced my life in a way that no pay-check or promotion could do.

It has literally brought some magic into my world and led me to connect with some incredible people. Similarly, our brand is flourishing as a result of our kind approach.

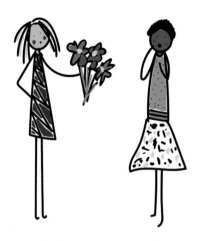

Kindness begins with learning to be compassionate towards yourself and this is often the hardest task of all. I have suffered from anxiety and low self-esteem in the past. I am not alone in this. But when I realised a few years ago that the pressure I felt was not coming from external sources, but actually from within myself, I was able to begin a process of growth. For me, that meant stopping comparing myself to others and seeking 'perfection' (whatever perfect means anyway) and I started to be kinder to myself; to lower my expectations and believe I was 'enough'. I began to focus my energy on appreciating the things I did have in my life and the things I achieved daily – no matter how small. I even said them out loud or wrote them down. I learned the power of kindly saying 'no' to things I didn't want to do – and this was one of the hardest challenges for me. I didn't go over my mistakes, I looked forward. I took things bit by bit, hour by hour, day by day. My life improved infinitely. I still return to this mantra when things feel overwhelming.

Having been on this journey, it was important to me that lots of practical ideas about how to bring self-compassion into your life are shared in this book. And they really work. I hope they help you too.

Jakki and I are so grateful to our friends, the experts, coaches, inspirational personalities and leaders in their fields who have shared words of kindness and offered tips that have enhanced their lives and improved the lives of others through the simple act of being kind. They have shown enormous kindness in doing this for us all.

This book is a true labour of love, and we hope it brings some magic into your life.

Kindness is your superpower – use it well.

Let us know how you get on!

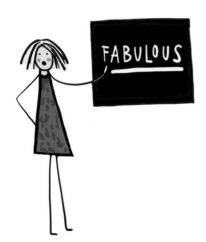

Love **Rosie**

Instagram
@rosiejnixon
@jakkidoodles

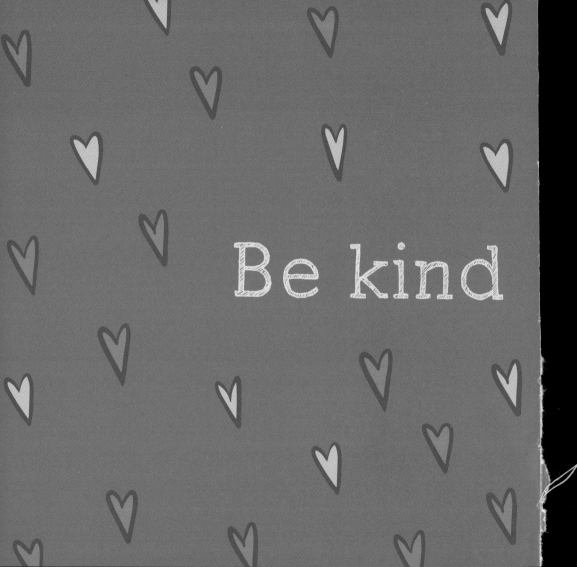

Be kind

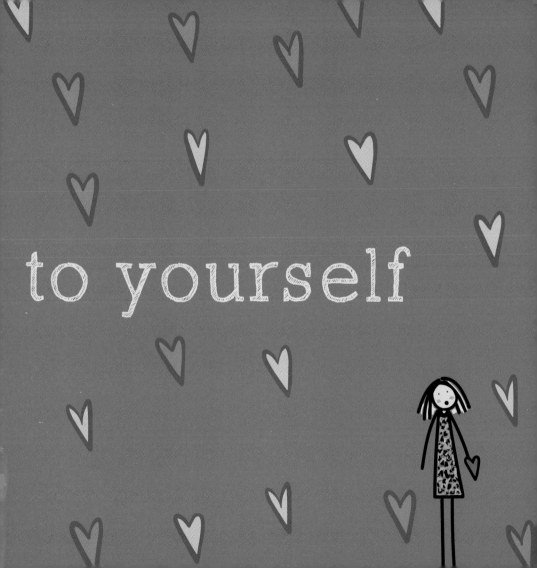

'Take care of my child
Take care of my wife
But I'm not so kind
To my restless mind'

Kelly Jones

Lyrics from 'Restless Mind',
from the album *Kind* by Stereophonics

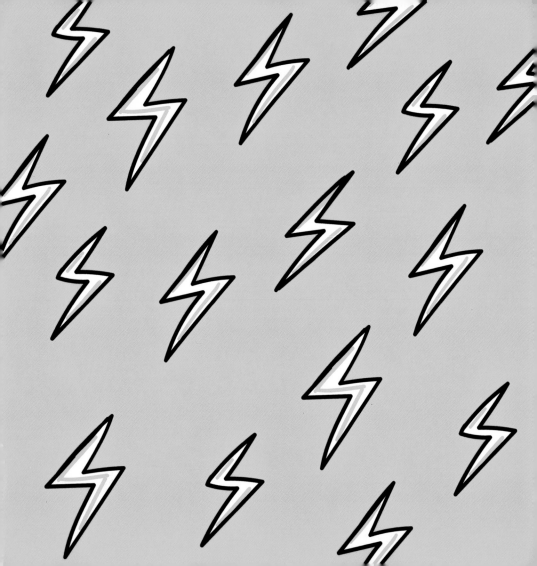

'We cannot think of being acceptable to others until we have first proven acceptable to ourselves' [1]

Malcolm X, Human rights activist

BE KIND:

Practise the following affirmations in the mirror:

♡ I love myself

♡ I am a beautiful person

♡ I accept myself

♡ I am talented

♡ I matter

♡ I am kind

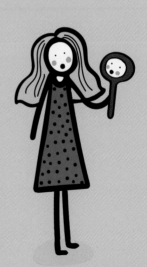

Self-compassion strategies

Self-compassion is showing warmth and kindness to yourself even in times of struggle, because you deserve to be treated with care. It is recognising that making mistakes is normal, and being kind to yourself when they occur.

BE KIND:

Start becoming more compassionate towards yourself by using these five strategies:

♥ Become aware of the times when you obtain a sense of self-worth from perfection or praise. Remind yourself that you are valued by your friends, partner or colleagues because of who you are, and not because you are faultless

♥ Find inspiration in other people's successes rather than negatively comparing yourself against them

♥ Practise gratitude. Appreciate the things you have in your life by writing them down, or simply by taking the time to notice them

♥ Treat yourself the way you would treat a friend

♥ Celebrate small wins. Take a moment to congratulate yourself for finishing a piece of work, remembering to do that job you've been putting off, or making time to go for a run

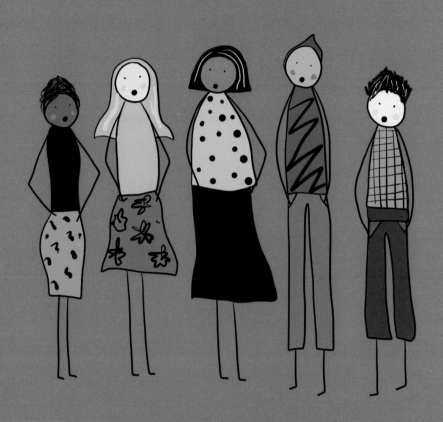

Kindness has to start within

'If we aren't kind to ourselves, we can't fully be kind to others. We might think we're being kind, but usually it'll come with resentment, burn-out or confusion down the line if we haven't started with kindness to ourselves. If we are kind to ourselves, we can set boundaries well with others, we can make decisions that come from the heart, and we can forgive and move on with more ease. Self-kindness means acknowledging our flaws, mistakes and past with acceptance so we don't drag them into the future. Kindness means doing the same with others in our lives. Kindness lives in the heart and connects us all.'

Fearne Cotton, Broadcaster and writer

Learn to love yourself

'From being a small child, we are encouraged to show kindness in the form of empathy and compassion to others, to be considerate, to be the friend who cares. And yet, we aren't taught to extend these feelings and services to ourselves. We tell ourselves it's selfish to think of ourselves first... which leads to hurtful self-talk and damaging beliefs. Kindness to others starts with being kind to ourselves; it is through our actions of self-love and self-care that we show our children the standard of love, care and kindness that they should expect to be treated with. We may have left our school days behind, but it is never too late to learn.'

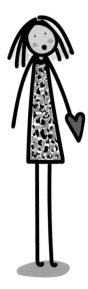

Andrea McLean,

Author, broadcaster and co-founder of www.thisgirlisonfire.com

BE KIND:

♥ Unlearn your negative self-talk. Would you talk to a friend the way you speak to yourself?

♥ Step away from those who don't show kindness towards you. Sure, everyone has a bad day, but if someone is consistently unkind to you the chances are they don't have your best interests at heart

♥ Remember 'Kindness to me...' doesn't just mean reflecting on what the word means to you. It can also mean showing kindness to yourself. Use it as your mantra to remind yourself that you deserve it

Soothe your soul with breathwork

Relaxing isn't easy, and often doesn't come naturally to us. Getting better at truly relaxing takes time and practice. It can start with something as simple as breathing. When was the last time you stopped everything and listened to your breath?

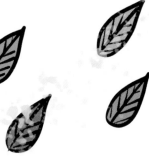

BE KIND:

- ♡ Focus on your breath

- ♡ Sit comfortably on a chair with both feet on the floor, or lie down

- ♥ Inhale slowly through your nose until you feel your stomach start to rise

- ♥ Hold your breath for a count of three

- ♥ Exhale slowly, letting your stomach fall

- ♥ Repeat this for a few minutes, allowing your breath to slow more and more with each inhale

THE WAY YOU SPEAK
TO YOURSELF MATTERS

'Whether your inner voice sounds like a best friend or a bully, it is with you every minute of your life and will impact your mental health. Many of us are highly self-critical until we feel that we have achieved enough. But that is like only watering a flower when it blooms. It is not conducive to good mental health, resilience and growth. Self-compassion is a necessity and one of the most vital tools we have for maintaining good mental wellbeing. We can't flourish without it.'

Dr Julie Smith,
Clinical psychologist (@drjuliesmith)

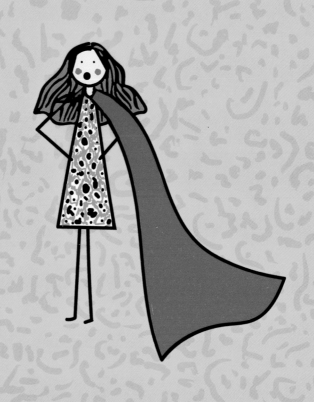

Be kind to yourself stretches

A trio of anti-stress stretches by **Karen Hauer**, professional dancer and *Strictly Come Dancing* star:

Neck rolls: Gently sit down cross-legged and get comfortable. Roll your neck eight times clockwise and eight times counter-clockwise, then bring your head back to the centre. We tend to hold a lot of emotional stress and anxiety on our shoulders and upper body, and this helps release it.

Cat and cow: Get onto all fours and find a neutral position where your back is flat, and your hands and knees are directly below your shoulders and hips respectively. Arch your back and push your head and neck to the sky, then push your back up and contract your stomach while pointing your head and neck to the floor. Repeat this eight times. Breathe naturally throughout. This is one of my favourites because it creates emotional balance, relieves stress and calms the mind as well as strengthens the spine.

Happy baby: Lie on your back, draw your knees into your chest wider than your ribcage with your legs at a ninety-degree angle and your ankles positioned over your knees. Grab on to the sides of your feet or your toes, and relax! This eases stress and anxiety, reduces lower back pain and opens the inner thighs, hips and groin.

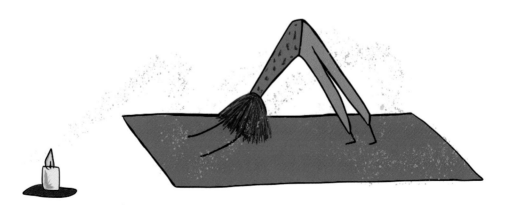

Self-care in ten simple steps

1. Sit with your thoughts for ten minutes and allow yourself to experience what you are feeling
2. Have a long soak in a bath
3. Go to bed early and read a book until your eyes feel heavy
4. Remember how far you have come
5. Compliment yourself verbally
6. Drink more water
7. Go for a walk
8. Wear sunscreen
9. Say goodbye to your inner critic
10. Cook your favourite meal

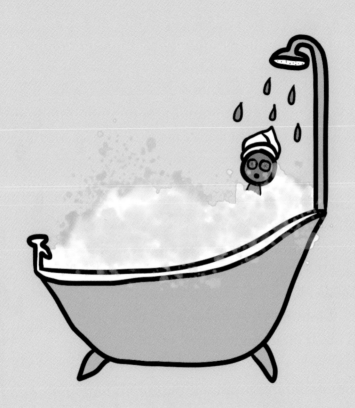

How to say 'no' with kindness

Often, people say 'yes' for fear of disappointing or hurting someone else. Most humans have a natural desire to be liked, but saying 'yes' all the time can be detrimental. Each time you say 'yes' to something you don't want to do (whether that's going to a party, taking on a new work commitment or going on a date with a someone you're not really interested in), you are using time that could be spent more wisely on more important things, like rest, hobbies, seeing friends and being with family. By politely saying 'no' to whatever it is someone is asking of you, you are actually saying 'yes' to what you truly want to be doing instead.

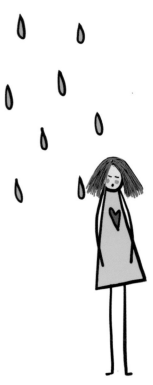

BE KIND:

5 ways to say 'no' nicely:

 When saying 'no', use your voice, face and body. Look the person in the eye and speak clearly and seriously while standing tall to project confidence and calm

 Repeat yourself if necessary, especially if people are used to you saying 'yes'

 Don't make excuses. You don't need to apologise for how you feel or what you want. It is better to say 'no' and feel slightly uncomfortable, than it is to say 'yes' and feel regret

 Use statements, not questions: 'I'm sorry but I'm not going to work any overtime this week' rather than 'Please can I not work any overtime this week?'

 Thank the other person for listening to your wishes

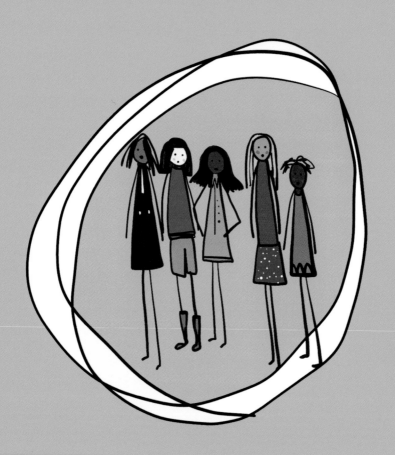

Socialise with kind people

- Walk away from negative thoughts and negative people

- Find a supportive community

- Open up to a friend or relative about how you really feel and encourage them to do the same

- If you don't leave a party feeling happy, ask yourself why

- Accept that you can't always gel with everyone

BELIEVE THINGS WILL
GET BETTER - THEY WILL

Research has shown that there is a strong
correlation between positive thinking and
overall life satisfaction, and that people who
visualise a better future for themselves are
more likely to live a fulfilled life.

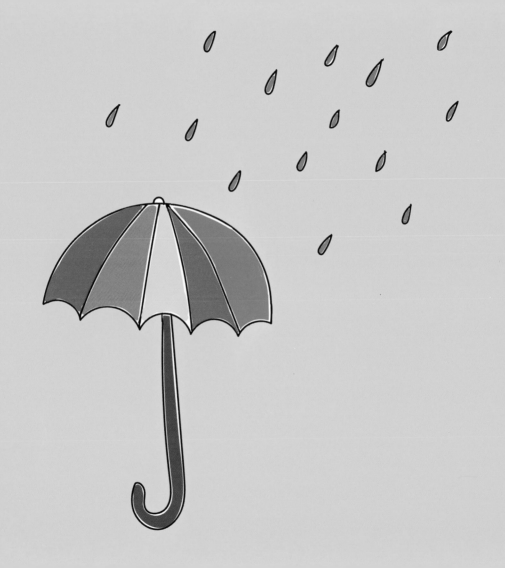

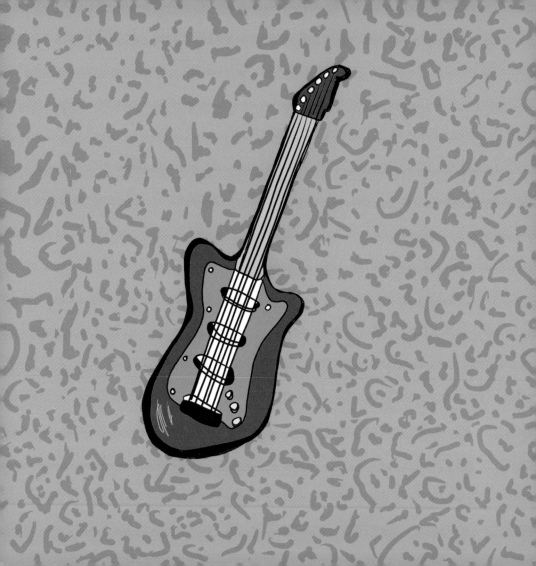

Use your greatest talent

'When I find myself facing challenges, what helps me to "keep keeping on" is being able to use my voice as an aid to others. Feeling needed and useful is a form of self-care. It is so edifying. To be able to sing to help raise money for a charity or provide entertainment to others reminds me of my purpose in life – to use music to enlighten and to uplift.

An act of kindness has real power, and the glow from the recipient of that act shines right back into your own soul.'

Beverley Knight MBE,

Singer and actress

Journal your feelings

Often, people feel less anxious after writing down their thoughts or concerns. Likewise, writing down what you are grateful for and your goals helps lift spirits and focus your efforts. Spend a week keeping a 'wellness diary' and see how it makes you feel.

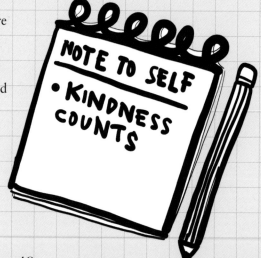

NOTE TO SELF
• KINDNESS COUNTS

BE KIND:

Here are some journaling tips:

- Keep your journal in a place that is cosy for you

- Make it a habit. Set a time to write, for example after waking up, while having breakfast or before bed, and stick to it every day

- Turn to your journal in moments of need. If you have had a difficult conversation, an argument, or are feeling particularly stressed or anxious, express how you are feeling in your journal

- Use your journal to reflect on what has happened. You can write about what you accomplished, things you are grateful for (or not so grateful for), and how you felt during the day

- Journal your goals: for the day, the week and the year ahead

- Tell your journal something you have been keeping from others. Is there a fear that is holding you back? Do you have an issue with someone you aren't ready to discuss yet? Write down what you would say if you were to have this conversation in person, and it might just help you get one step closer to overcoming these obstacles

Have a digital detox

'Don't give too much of yourself to your online profile. Look after yourself first, and only share what you are comfortable with.'

Natalie Pinkham,

Television presenter and podcaster

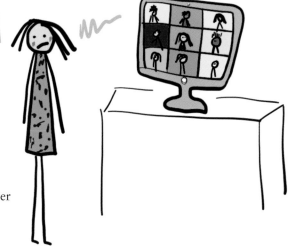

BE KIND:

♥ Unfollow social media accounts that leave you feeling negative about yourself

♥ Turn off push notifications

♥ Unsubscribe to emails you receive from a list that you don't want to be on

♥ Buy an alarm clock, so your phone isn't the first thing you look at when you wake up

♥ Establish a 'No Phone Zone' at the dinner table and in bed

♥ Take a break from social media for a week and see how it makes you feel

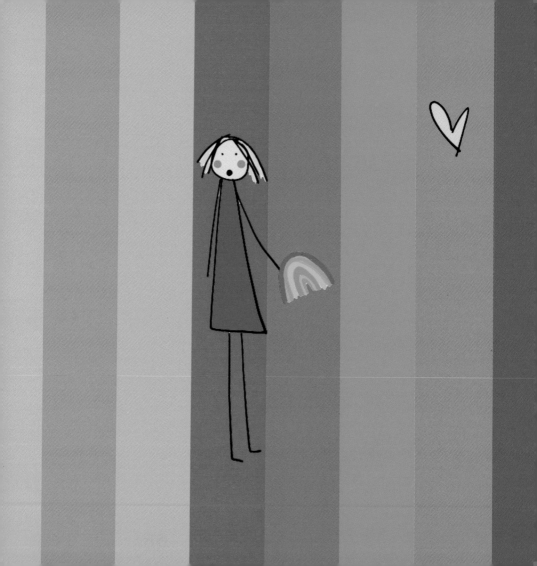

FOCUS ON THE POSITIVES

'I think we can be quick to give ourselves negative feedback. Maybe it's human nature, but we need to change that mentality. We must be kinder to ourselves and to others – so much good can come from an act of kindness. It's something we need to instil in children – kindness from a young age will make the future so much brighter.'

Alex Scott MBE,

Sports presenter and
ex-England football captain

Change your mindset

Often our minds only focus on the anxiety-inducing 'what ifs':

What if I have a horrible time?

What if I fail?

What if everyone laughs at me?

It is important to remember that there is also a different, kinder, way to think:

What if I succeed?

What if I have the best night of my life?

What if it helps me grow?

Making an effort to change your inner monologue might, in turn, change your life.

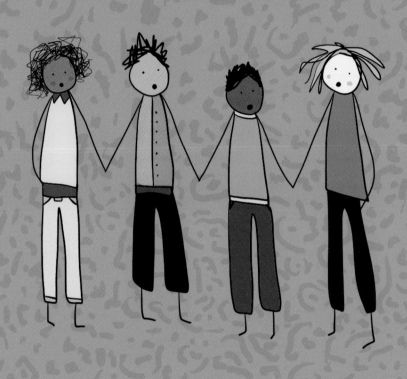

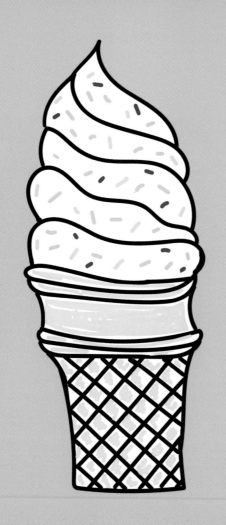

Have a kind night in

The next time Friday evening comes around, treat yourself to the ultimate night in. Here are some tips to make it extra kind:

⭐ Comfort is critical, so make sure you've got plenty of cushions and blankets (or even duvets). Draw the curtains, light some candles and get cosy

⭐ Put on your favourite loungewear

⭐ Buying a fancy tub of ice cream can get a bit pricey, so why not make your own ice cream concoction? Top what you already have in the freezer with crushed biscuits, nuts, chocolate or fruit. Or just invest in your favourite treat

⭐ Re-watch a film or TV series that you love, perhaps something you watched as a child or teenager, and enjoy a wave of nostalgia as you meet your favourite characters again

⭐ If you have company, keep it simple and play some games

⭐ Attempt to learn a new card game together

Kindness is good for you

Alongside physical exercise, being kind is one of the most important things you can do for your cardiovascular health. The hormone oxytocin is vital for your heart and can be generated through showing compassion and warmth to others.

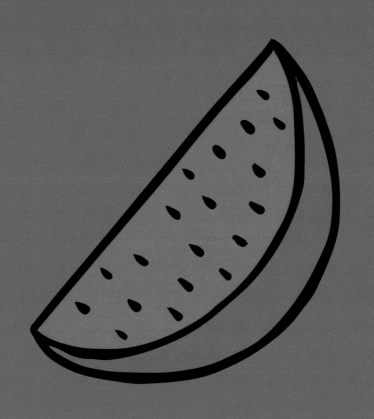

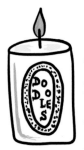

'Kindness, to me, means being authentic, open and happy. There is a quote that stays with me, it says: "Every act of kindness is a sadaqa (charity)". In terms of being kind to myself, I have learned along the way in the fashion industry not to beat myself up for every mistake I've made. Being true to who you are is being kind to yourself and this is a point I'd really like to drive home to the women of minorities, not just in modelling, but in all fields of work.'

Ikram Abdi Omar,

Fashion model and champion of greater minority representation

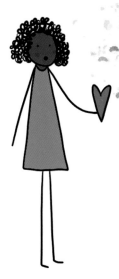

KINDNESS NEEDS
YOU TO BE PRESENT

'I focus on taking small pleasures from everyday life,
whether that's taking the first sip of your coffee in the
morning, or watching the sun rise. Enjoy those moments,
and be grateful to have them.'

Dermot O'Leary,
Television and radio host and author

BE KIND:

♥ Think about the next minute, the next hour, today

♥ Notice three things in nature that are beautiful around you. Really look at them and appreciate them

♥ Don't get lost in the depths of 'what ifs'

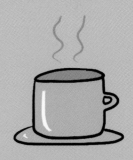

Self-care and the great outdoors

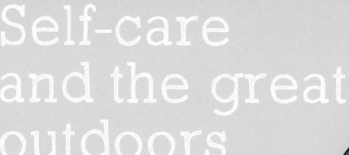

Spending time in green spaces has been found to benefit your mental and physical wellbeing.
This can be achieved in a number of ways:

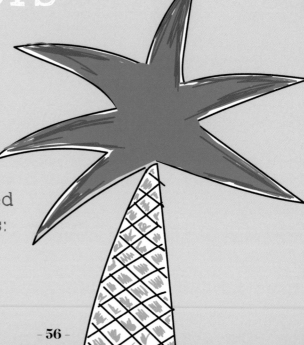

- Grow your own food, flowers or house plants

- Exercise outdoors

- Spend time with animals

- Arrange a comfortable place to sit by a window where you can look at trees or the sky

- Have your lunch break outside rather than eating at your desk

- Go camping

- Watch the stars

- Hug a tree

15 kind lessons worth learning:

1. There's a certain ebb and flow to life. Happiness won't be constant and that's OK

2. People's lives aren't always as perfect as their social media suggests

3. Friendships come and go

4. It's OK to take a sick day for your mental health

5. Trust your gut, it's usually right

6. Make time for your hobbies

7   We all need to ask for help sometimes

8   It's human nature to make mistakes

9   How you speak to yourself matters

10   Stand up for the things you believe in

11   You are stronger than you think

12   Comparing yourself to others won't lead to happiness

13   Even the most confident people struggle with insecurity

14   Embrace change as opportunity

15   All you can do is your best, and your best is truly enough

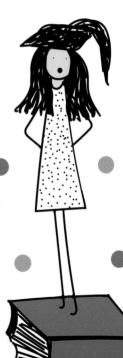

'You don't have to continually improve yourself to love yourself. Love is not something you only deserve if you reach a goal. The world is a world of pressure but don't let it squeeze your self-compassion. You were born worthy of love and you remain worthy of love. Be kind to yourself.'

Matt Haig,

Author and mental health advocate

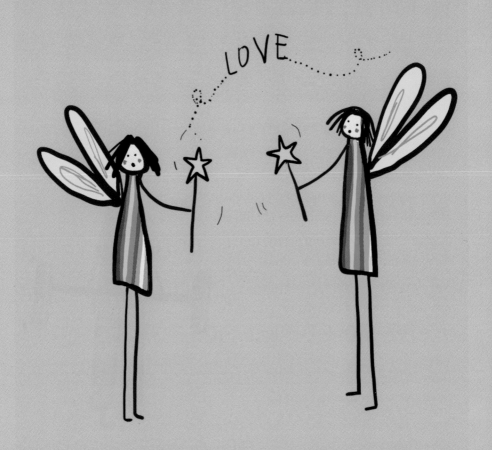

Kindness and motherhood

'As mothers, we often question our actions, constantly asking ourselves if we're doing a good enough job. I am often guilty of speaking unkindly to myself, with a little critic who sits on my shoulder and talks to me about all sorts of negative things, I've realised I rarely think anything kind about myself. Here is a way to mindfully remind ourselves how to think and speak kindly.'

Izzy Judd,

Mindfulness advocate and author

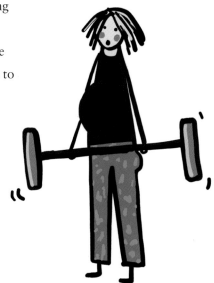

IZZY'S KINDNESS INTENTION

Start the day with an affirmation to remind
yourself to be kind about yourself and to others:

'Today I choose to think kindly
about myself.'

'Today I will let a friend know how much
happiness they bring to my life.'

'Today I choose to do something
kind for myself.'

10 things to give up, to be kind to yourself

1. The need for control or perfection
2. Fearing change
3. Overthinking
4. Ignoring your intuition
5. Gossiping
6. Negative self-attitude
7. Trying to please everyone
8. Living in the past
9. Indecisiveness
10. Running from problems that need fixing

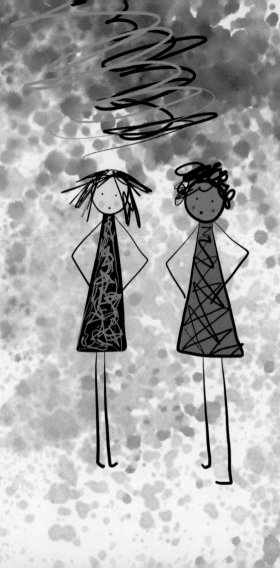

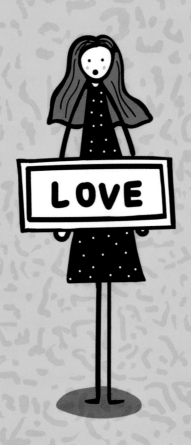

Kindness is attractive

A study by the *Journal of Personality* spoke to 2,700 people from five different countries about what they most look for in a potential partner. Out of physical attractiveness, humour, financial prospects, creativity and many other attributes, it was kindness that proved most important.

'An attractive human being is one with a kind heart, a listening ear, loving words and a beautiful soul. A beautiful soul is one that radiates kindness, love and compassion and mesmerises all who come within its path. Be a beautiful soul and let kindness be your trademark.'

Sheela Mackintosh-Stewart,

Family lawyer

Define yourself as 'kind'

'On occasion, you will be asked to describe yourself in three words. The first word that springs into my mind is "kind". Now this kindness might merely be a subconscious goal of mine, or perhaps rather a genuine attribute that I carry around, I do hope that my friends and family would confirm the latter! Simply that I dare to utter the K word when defining myself makes me feel incredibly proud.

I assume this is because I haven't always been kind to everyone. I spent a decade being ghastly to myself when I was suffering with severe acne.

Now, I do still suffer with my skin, but over time I've learned that the real joy of kindness only takes effect when you are kind to absolutely everyone, and that must include yourself.

I smile now when I look in the mirror; my acne and my scars are a part of me and I am not ashamed anymore. Without my dedication to being kind I do wonder whether this desperately important shift would have ever taken place.

Kindness makes the world go round, these small acts are the sum of how we humans feel loved, contented and is the most valuable currency we have.'

Georgia Toffolo,

Television and media personality and author

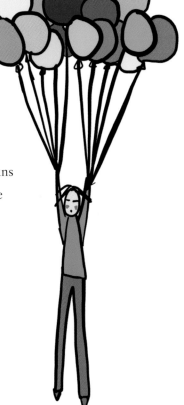

YOU

 Are here for a reason

 Are incredible for getting through
tough times

 Are not defined by others, or by the past

 Are worthy of love, success and happiness

 Are more than enough

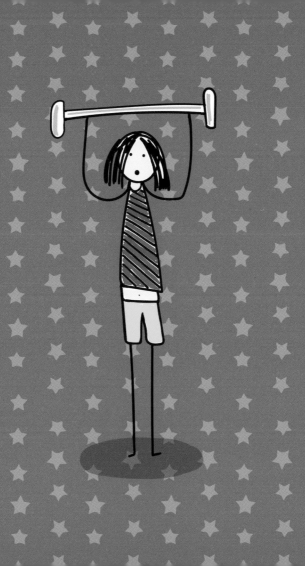

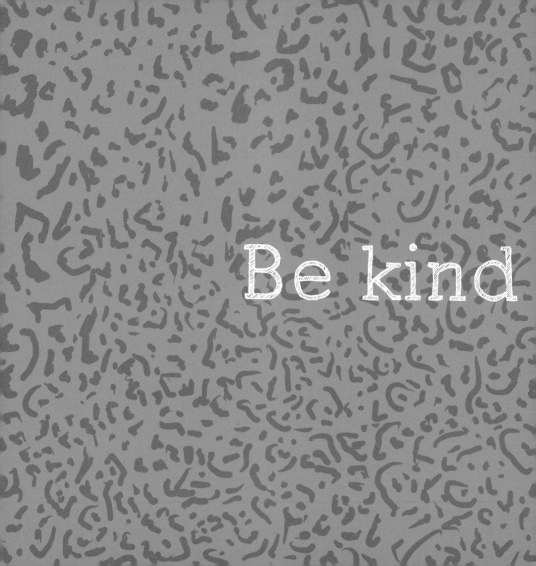

Be kind

to others

'Share the gift of kindness. How you make others feel is a choice. Choose to be kind, even to the unkind ones. There is real power in that.'

Holly Willoughby,

Television presenter

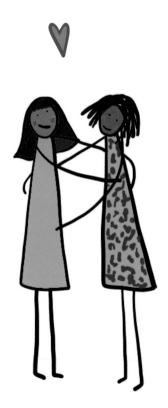

BE KIND:

Select from the messages below and text them to the people who light up your world

I just want you to know, I'm so grateful to have you in my life.

I was just thinking of you and wanted to say hello.

I know you've been working so hard recently. Make sure you're getting enough sleep!

Life is so much better with you in it.

Sending you positive vibes! I'm here if you ever need to talk.

Missing you! Tell me when you're next free.

Just checking in – how have you been doing?

Do you remember when we did _____ together?! Let's meet up soon!

Pay someone a compliment

'You never know how much something so simple as genuinely complimenting an outfit you admire can set someone off on a more positive path for the rest of their day.

I know this to be true from experience. For me, being a somewhat unusual dresser, getting random insults shouted at me is the norm. But those times when people stopped and genuinely complimented my look really gave me a positive strut in my step for the rest of the day. It's not about a need to be complimented, it's about knowing that amongst the sea of hate there are people out there who appreciate your existence. To those people who said nice things, I don't think you even realised the power you gave me.

I try not to hold anything against rude and mean people either. You never know what someone's going through and their reasons for behaving in such a way. It's with this mindset I try to live my life. Treat everybody with friendliness and kindness, you don't know how much they need it.'

Jamie Campbell, Drag queen

BE KIND:

Lift someone's spirits today by giving them one of the following compliments:

You are one of the strongest people I know.

You are beautiful inside and out.

You inspire me.

You're such a good friend.

I am so glad we met.

I love spending time with you.

You have the best laugh.

I really appreciate everything you do.

Your point of view is so refreshing.

Thanks for always being there for me.

You are so creative.

You are an incredible human, I'm lucky to know you.

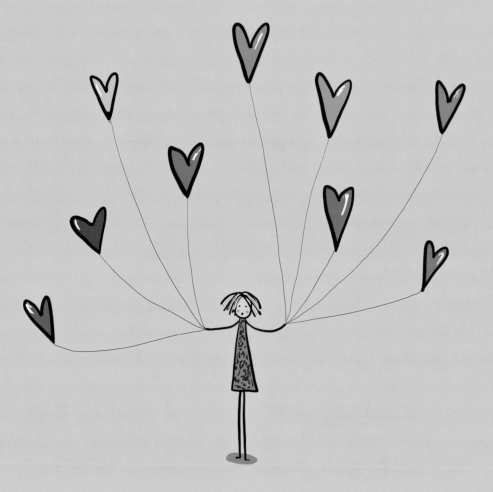

'My father used to say: "When you meet someone who is not wearing a smile, give them one of yours". That is how I live my life.'

Nancy Durrell McKenna,

Photographer, film-maker and founder director of SafeHands

Spread the joy of kindness

When you're kind to someone, it's not just that person that feels the benefit. Any small act of kindness you perform has a ripple effect onto others. The person you are kind to will likely go on to be kind to five other people. Those five people will go on to show kindness to five more and so on.

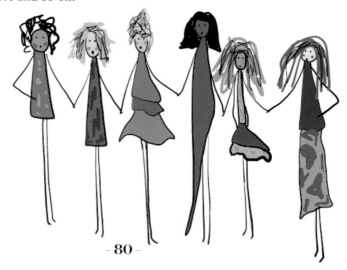

BE KIND:

♥ Hold the door open for someone

♥ Deliver a handwritten note to an elderly neighbour to check whether they need anything

♥ Tell someone you're proud of them

♥ Offer a hug

♥ Tag a friend in a post that will make them smile

♥ Start a conversation by asking: 'Tell me about your weekend.' Give your full, undivided attention without waiting to talk about yourself

Kind cooking

'My favourite way to show my appreciation for someone is to make them something delicious. Homemade is the best as it's love and kindness straight from my kitchen to their stomach (and hopefully hearts!).

Eating these chocolate nut butter truffles has got to be one of life's true happy moments. So much so that when I was first testing this recipe five years ago, they were nicknamed the Happiness Balls. Share the extras with someone else, and the happiness factor goes through the roof!

The toppings can be adapted so as to best please the receiver. And if you can keep an eye out for the Fairtrade symbol on some of the ingredients, you'll be using your purchasing power for the greater global good and supporting farmers across the world to earn a fair wage.'

Melissa Hemsley, Chef, author and sustainability champion

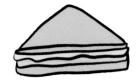

Happiness Balls

10 minutes to make, 1-2 hours in the freezer to set, then 10 more minutes to roll!

Ingredients:
4 tbsp coconut oil
4 tbsp maple syrup
6 tbsp cocoa powder (look for Fairtrade)
8 tbsp nut butter of your choice (e.g. cashew, peanut, almond)
Pinch of sea salt

Topping Ideas:
2 tbsp cocoa powder
2 tbsp desiccated coconut
2 tbsp finely-chopped pistachios or hazelnuts
2 tbsp freeze-dried raspberries or strawberries

Method:

1. Melt the coconut oil in a medium saucepan, then add the maple syrup, cocoa powder, nut butter and sea salt. Stir to combine.

2. Pour into a wide heatproof shallow dish. The wider the dish, the faster it will cool.

3. Place in the fridge to set for 1–2 hours. Alternatively, you can speed up the process by placing in the freezer for an hour or so.

4. When the mixture has set, use a tablespoon and dry hands to form it into twenty 2cm balls. If they're too sticky, put them back in the fridge or freezer to harden some more.

5. Place the toppings in different bowls and roll each ball in the topping until covered on all sides. Enjoy immediately, store in the fridge or give to friends, family or neighbours!

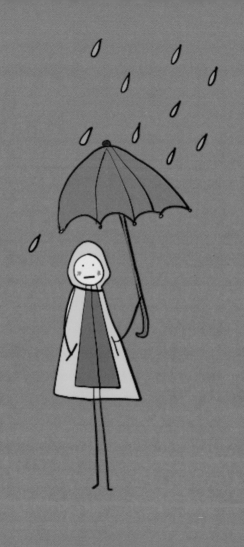

How to have a kind conversation

Truly listening to someone requires active engagement. Here's how to achieve that:

 Make sure you put your phone away

 Use your body language to show that you're listening. Uncross your arms, lean slightly forwards, make eye contact

 Pay attention to the speaker's facial expressions and body language, which can convey more emotions than their words

 Don't interrupt

 Ask open-ended questions

 Use minimal encouragers, such as 'mmm', 'I see', 'OK', 'yes', or nodding and facial expressions to show the person you hear them, and prompt them to continue talking

 Carefully consider your response before speaking. Meaningful conversations often take time

Make kindness your mindset

'To me, kindness is taking the time to consider other people with empathy and understanding.'

Katie Piper,

Television presenter and confidence coach

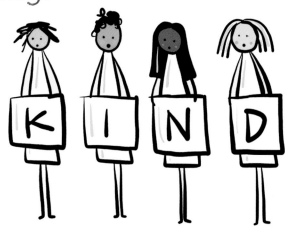

BE KIND:

Here are Katie's little acts of kindness:

♥ Say good morning to a stranger. This might catch them off guard, but it's a lovely act of kindness

♥ If you see someone with heavy suitcases, or struggling to carry a pushchair up some stairs, stop and offer to help them

♥ Let an old teacher know that they inspired you, or a boss who helped you progress in your career, by writing them a card. Receiving a handwritten letter will brighten someone's day

♥ Always, always, always pass a good book along on to somebody else

♥ Follow the one-in, one-out rule: every time you buy or receive a new item of clothing, give an old one away. You could drop it at a charity shop or shelter, or gift it to someone you know – something you know they will like and enjoy

'One of the biggest challenges you face in sport is whether to be fair and kind. Not only to yourself but to your competitors. If you can master that art, you will always be a winner.'

Denise Lewis OBE,
Sports presenter and Olympic track and field gold medalist

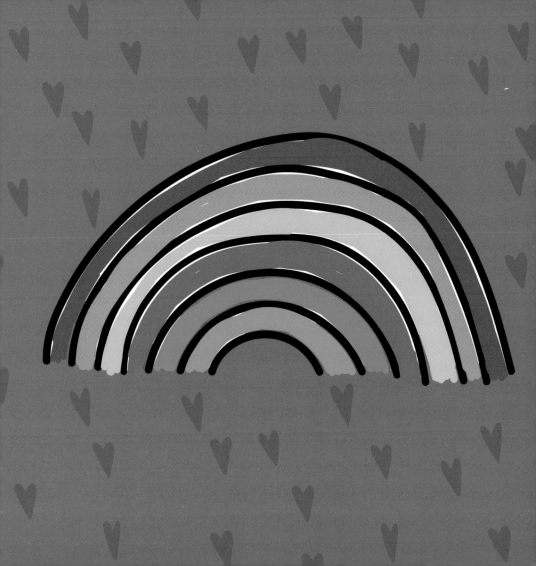

Be kind to strangers

'Not much in life is free but kindness is, and the richest person on earth can't buy it cos it's free! So give it out! Give it to everyone. Lend everyone your kind cos one day you might need a bit of kind yourself. It takes as much or as little time as you want to give it and everyone has it. Just takes a little thought. And the thought is all that counts!'

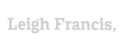

Leigh Francis,

Comedian, actor and writer

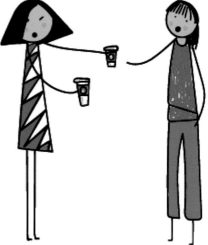

BE KIND:

 Smile at a person in the street

 Thank your taxi or bus driver and mean it

 Ask someone how their day is going

 Tell someone that you like their outfit

 Compliment the next person who serves you in a shop, cafe or restaurant, smile and tell them you hope they have a blessed day

 Tell a shop manager what a great job their employee is doing

 Strike up a conversation with someone while you're waiting in a shop or at a train station; it might be the first conversation they have had all day

 Buy a coffee for the person behind you in the queue

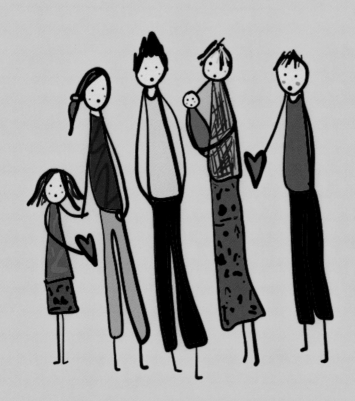

KINDNESS
CREATES CALM

Kindness has been found to reduce anxiety in
those who perform kind acts.[2]

Connecting with kindness

Keeping in touch with friends and relatives on a regular basis can be difficult. Here are some easy ideas to ensure you don't go months on end without seeing one another:

- Arrange a time each week to work out together. FaceTime while doing yoga or a home workout, or meet in person for a run, walk or swim

- Commit to watching a TV series together. Meet up each week to watch the latest episode or watch from your own homes while on a video call. You could even call each other after the show to discuss it

- Run your errands together! Chances are that you both have parcels to post, or a food shop to do, so agree to do them together. If you can't do it in person, plug in your headphones or airpods and catch up on the phone while grabbing your shopping

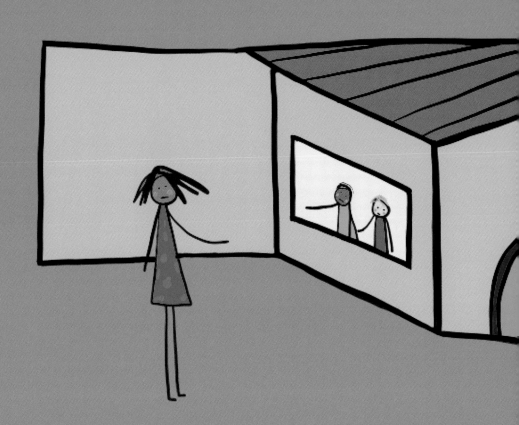

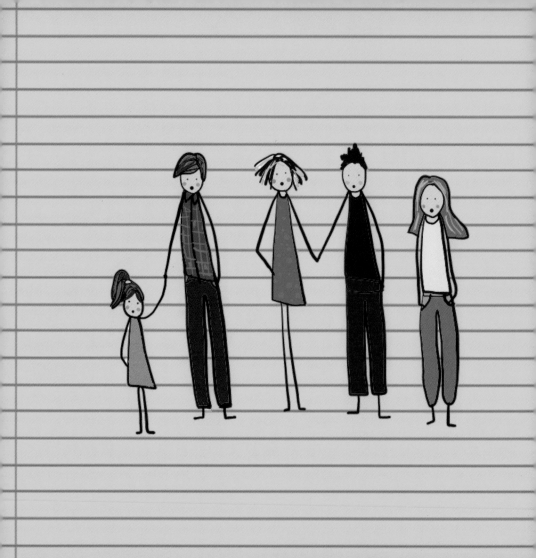

Subtle ways to show appreciation for your friends and family

Kindness isn't about grand gestures. Here are some simple ways to show someone how much you care:

 Wear or use a gift they gave you when you next see them

 Show them you value their opinion by asking for their advice

 Make time for them

 Offer to do something you know they don't enjoy, like washing up or mowing the lawn

 Show an interest in something they are passionate about

 Ask them to teach you something – you get to develop, and they feel as though their knowledge is appreciated

 Be on time (or early) when you see them to demonstrate how important they are to you

How to show kindness in your relationships

 Pay attention. If your partner, parent or friend tells you they have had a bad day, say more than 'I'm sorry about that'. Take the time to sit with them and listen to what has happened.

 If they are eager to tell you about a new hobby, ask questions and show them that because it is something they care about, you care about it, too. Even if it doesn't interest you!

 Let it go. Have they put your laundry in the wrong drawer, or forgotten to put the dishwasher on? Remind yourself that criticising will only make their day worse, and not actually resolve the issue. Move on.

Be inclusive. Involve them in as many decisions as you can, so that they feel you are truly a team.

 When someone has done something that makes you angry, it's often hard to remain calm and resolve the problem with kindness. If necessary, tell them you need some time to think or calm down before discussing what has happened. When you do talk about it with them, remember that your goal is not to 'win' the argument, but to reach an outcome where you both feel OK.

 Be their strength. Notice where they have weaknesses and fill in the gaps. If you notice they are tired, take on some of the housework they usually do. If they have trouble standing up for themselves, help them to write an assertive email or prepare for a conversation.

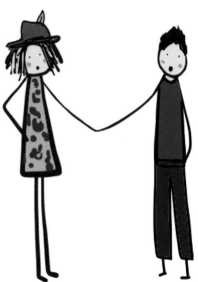

Breaking up
with kindness

'The end of a relationship is always difficult – but this is actually a perfect opportunity to make the effort to be kind. First and foremost, be kind to yourself. This will give you a greater capacity to be kind to others. Accepting that things don't always go according to plan, and following the necessary grieving process, will help you develop a refined sense of self-awareness.

By removing yourself from your immediate personal experience, looking at the events from the outside, you will be able to put yourself in your ex's shoes more easily. This empathy is absolutely critical to being kind.

Taking a bird's eye view of the situation will help you to communicate calmly and openly while considering the needs and views of others. This will encourage your ex to reciprocate. Being kind isn't always easy when you're navigating a break-up, but it will make a positive difference throughout the process and into the next chapter of your lives.'

Bec Jones, Divorce coach

'I think it all boils down to this: life is much more fun when you're wrapped in a kindness quilt, than when you're trapped in the spikes of cruelty.'

Bryony Gordon,

Author and journalist

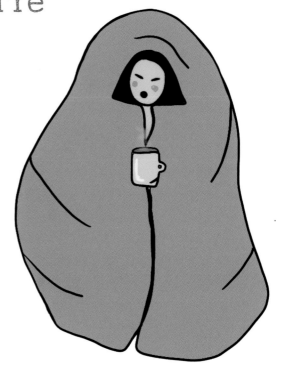

'Kindness has always been
the main conversation in our
house; something I am constantly
discussing with my children.
For us, it is about taking time
out to understand people: their
differences, their needs, their
worries, being considerate
and listening. A small act
of kindness could change
someone's life.'

Emma Bunton,

Singer, songwriter and actress

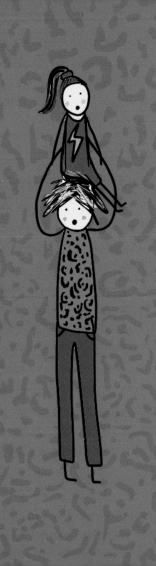

How to show kindness to children

 Speak to them the way you would an adult. Children have lots to say, so listening to their ideas and engaging in an active conversation will demonstrate that you value their opinions.

 Get on their level. If possible, kneel or sit so that you are at eye level with them when you are having conversations. This is much less intimidating for little ones, and will encourage them to be more open with you.

 Don't underestimate them. Children are much more capable than you might think, and are able to comprehend complex ideas, as well as handle important tasks and jobs. Give them responsibilities to make them feel valued, and talk to them about normal, everyday issues without babying them.

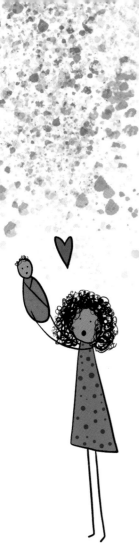

⭐ Support their passions. You might have outgrown fairies, dinosaurs or fire engines years ago, but try your best to be enthusiastic about the things that they are interested in. Involving yourself in their play will help them realise their interests and also develop their skills to play collaboratively with other children.

⭐ Don't put pressure on them. A child who is under pressure is more likely to grow up with increased feelings of anxiety. Let them grow at their own pace.

'My parents taught me about the importance of qualities like kindness, respect and honesty, and I realise how central values like these have been to me throughout my life. That is why William and I want to teach our little children just how important these things are as they grow up. In my view, it is just as important as excelling at maths or sport.'[3]

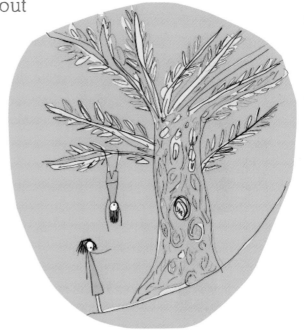

The Duchess of Cambridge

BE KIND:

Promote kindness in children by following the below steps:

 Encourage children to talk about the kind things they have done for others during their day

 Model kind behaviour

 Play 'let's pretend' games to practise being kind. Comfort their teddy who's hurt himself, or pretend teddy needs to tidy their room and help him do it. This will help children develop their ability to view life from the perspective of others and develop their social and emotional intelligence

 Make helping a family affair – get children involved in baking cakes to deliver to neighbours, tidying away the dishes or writing cards to tell relatives you are thinking of them

 Help children spot kindness in their community. Whenever you go to the park, notice kind acts that might be happening and draw your child's attention to them, such as someone putting their litter in a bin, or someone helping another person cross the road, and show them that you're willing to do the same!

Modelling kind behaviour to children

'To be kind is the ultimate strength. Genuine kindness can only come when we have learned what it is to be kind to ourselves. This is why parenting is so crucial. When we know kindness we are easily able to extend expressions of kindness to others. So, first, be kind to yourself. When we practise self-care, we can more easily achieve what we call "emotional regulation", or what I call "wise owl thinking". It allows us as parents to keep calm in the face of the squabbles and shouts. Rather than resorting to shouting, we are able to remain calm and kind and use our words to express how we feel – so our children are much more likely to model that behaviour in turn. Teaching our children how to tap into their "wise owl" brain, helps them to be kind to others, to use words to resolve their issues (rather than means!), to maintain a "big picture" perspective throughout their lives, and ultimately to empathise with others.

Being empathetic could be considered the true source of kindness. When our children are able to step into the shoes of another – to consider how another child or person might be feeling and consider their actions towards them as a result, that, to me, is being kind.'

Kate Silverton,

Presenter, author and
child psychology expert

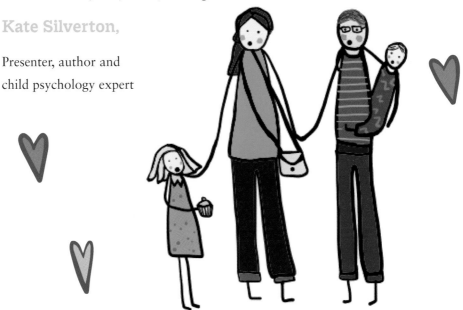

Kindness at work

Being compassionate to others increases your own confidence and productivity, so spreading kindness in your office will help you and others become more efficient at work.

'Kindness is not complicated but over the years it has been translated, especially in business, as a weakness. Being kind is what I call a "simple superpower"; we all have it but not everyone uses it. As a new CEO it encapsulates making time for my team, listening to them about what they want and need and making changes that create a workplace that everyone loves. I can only do this if I am kind to myself first, and I am unapologetically

selfish in this pursuit. In order to be kind to people, you must be outrageously kind to yourself first. You'll have more than enough empathy, compassion and space to give to others.'

Natalie Campbell, CEO and motivational speaker

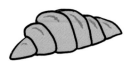

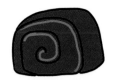

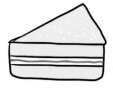

BE KIND:

How to cultivate kindness in your office:

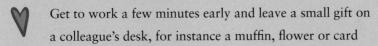

Get to work a few minutes early and leave a small gift on a colleague's desk, for instance a muffin, flower or card

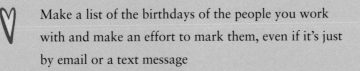

Make a list of the birthdays of the people you work with and make an effort to mark them, even if it's just by email or a text message

Offer to buy lunch or a coffee for your direct report on a day when they appear too busy to get it themselves

Bake a cake and bring it to the office for everyone to share

Acknowledge somebody's talent or skill, and tell them you appreciate them

Spend time getting to know new employees by asking about their passions outside of work

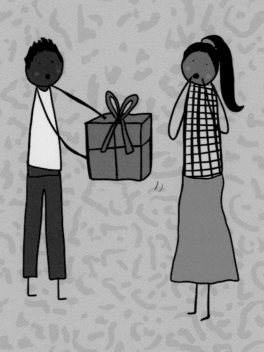

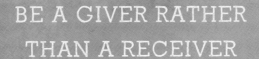

BE A GIVER RATHER
THAN A RECEIVER

Giving to others has been found to reduce
blood pressure and alleviate pain. This is
because regions of the brain that react to
painful stimulation appear to be deactivated
by the experience of giving.

'When I think of the people that mean the most to me, they all have one thing in common: they are genuinely kind. When they ask "how are you" they really want to know the answer, and always seem to sense when you need a hug or some reassurance. I don't think we should ever underestimate the power of even the smallest act of kindness because it can make all the difference in the world.

I've been the stranger who pays for a coffee when someone has forgotten their purse or given up my seat on the bus or tube when I see a woman struggling with shopping or looking tired and exhausted. I try to be the friend or colleague at work who says how terrific someone is looking and that I love their outfit, because it can really make their day.

I think it's a good idea to wake up in the morning with the mindset that you are going to be kind, big-hearted, and also try your best to find something positive even when things are at their toughest and most difficult.

When you give out a little bit of kindness it comes back to you a hundred-fold, and you will feel lighter and happier. I know I do.'

Lorraine Kelly,

Television presenter

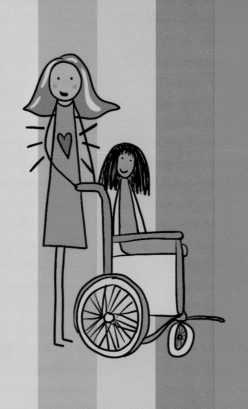

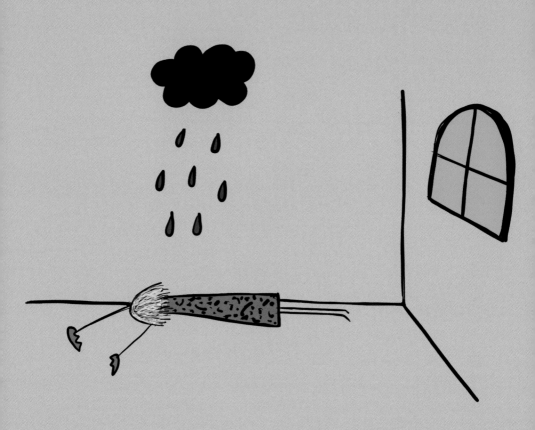

How to support someone struggling right now:

1. Get informed – educate yourself on their condition or situation to better understand them
2. Let them talk and listen empathetically without judgement; let them share as much or as little as they want and let them know you're there for them
3. Ask them what you can do to help them
4. Encourage them to accept help if they need it. Offer to go with them to appointments/the doctor/food shopping, and remind them to take care of themselves
5. Be patient with them
6. Check in on them frequently so they know they're not alone
7. Know your own limits: don't burn yourself out helping someone. Make sure to take time for yourself and your own mental health, too

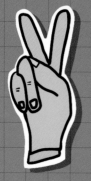

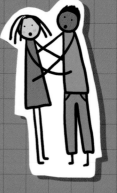

Be kind

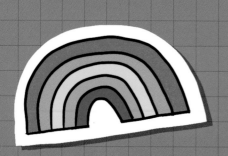

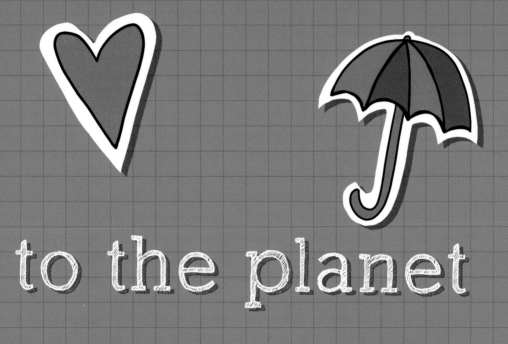

to the planet

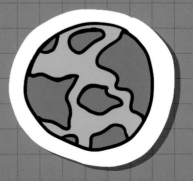

'Be kind whenever possible. It is always possible.'[4]

The 14th Dalai Lama

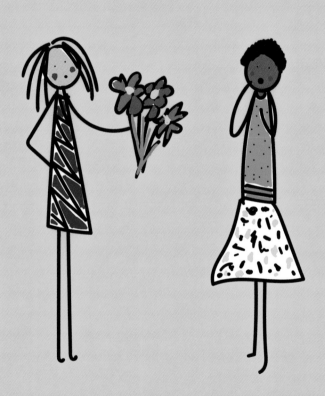

Kindness in the community

'Do your little bit of good where you are; it's those little bits of good put together that overwhelm the world.' [5]

Desmond Tutu,

Human rights activist

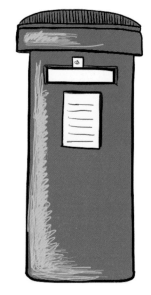

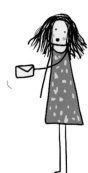

BE KIND:

♡ Take a bag with you when you go out and collect any litter you see today

♡ Support a local business instead of purchasing things online

♡ Donate to a charity, or set up regular monthly donations if you're able to

♡ Tip your waiter

♡ Give blood

♡ Respect people's pronouns

'Kindness is remembering, kindness is loyalty, kindness is friendship, and kindness is never forgetting who has been there through thick and thin. Through good days, bad days, rainy days. Kindness can be a superpower. All we can do is lead by example. The game I have is, the more cruel people are, the more I smile. And I will keep smiling.'

The Duchess of York

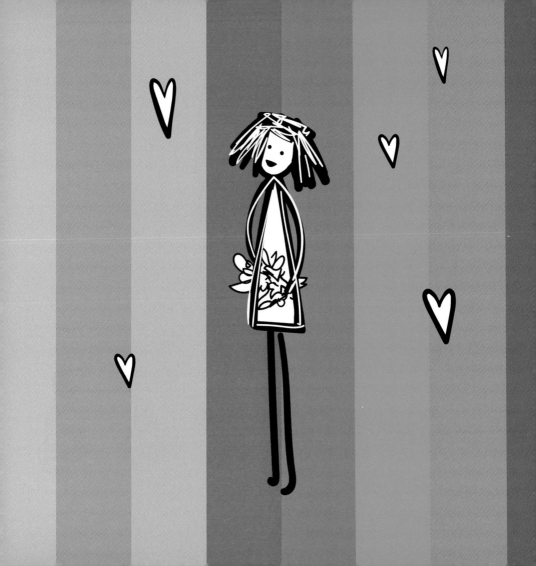

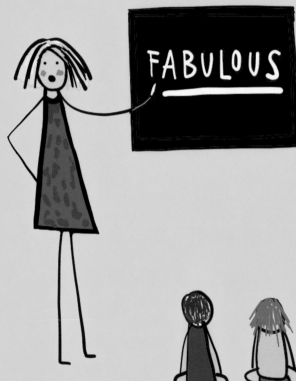
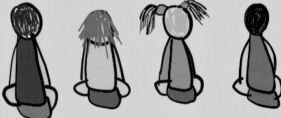

How to be more empathetic

Empathy is an emotional engine that gives purpose and adds meaning and joy to our acts of kindness. We often think of empathy as something a person either 'has' or 'doesn't have', but empathy is a skill that can be developed. Here are some ideas:

 Spend time cultivating friendships with people who have different values and beliefs to yourself. Building deep personal connections with people who might not think the same things as you will improve your empathy

 Attend someone else's place of worship for a few weeks and encourage them to attend yours

 Work for a community project where you'll meet people you wouldn't ordinarily socialise with

 Volunteer for a charity: not only will it build your confidence and help you develop your skills, you'll learn from people with backgrounds that differ to yours and be given the satisfaction of feeling like you're helping in some small way

There is no solution without kindness

'Whether it's raising my children or wondering whether it's possible to steer our troubled world away from the abyss – there is no solution without kindness.

Kindness is a willingness to approach one another in loving good faith, whether those people are strangers or the ones we know most intimately.

My own program of recovery has shown me that it's often easier to be kind to those with whom there is little at stake, a drug addict that you'll never see again, whereas it's harder to be kind to your partner, and sometimes impossible to be kind to yourself. I have been shown that when I believe that there is nothing to get, that ultimately everyone you encounter in life is worthy of kindness, they were born, they will die, then I can live in peace. This simple word, when used in the form of raising your children or saving our world, could be the key to changes we need to make.'

Russell Brand, Comedian, actor, writer and activist

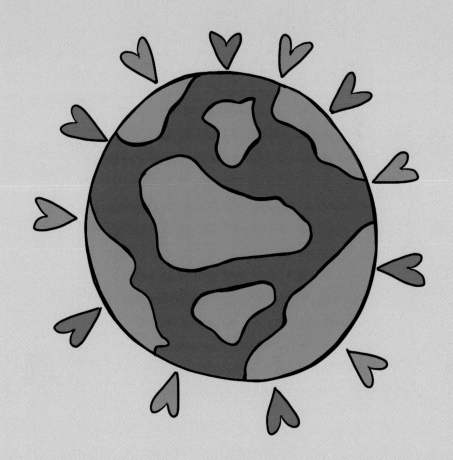

How to be a better feminist

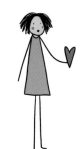

1. Read up. Gather a global perspective of women's struggles by educating yourself on the experiences of women across the globe. This will help you understand your privilege, whether it's through class, race, gender or sexuality

2. Ask for what you deserve, and make sure the other women around you do the same. If you feel as though you deserve a pay rise, stand tall and confidently present your manager with evidence of the contribution you make. Encourage other women to realise their worth and make sure they aren't selling themselves short

3. Advocate for women's rights. Attend conferences happening near you, get involved with campaigns or charities that support women, or offer your own skills to tutor teenage girls who need mentoring

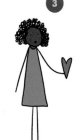

4 Support female entrepreneurs. Buy from their businesses and promote their products through your own platforms. If you are able to, invest in their business to help them grow

5 Teach your children to be feminists. Avoid gendered toys and if your daughter, niece, grandchild or godchild wants to play football, get outside and play with her

6 Encourage boys to show their emotions and allow them to express themselves in any way they wish

7 Teach children about consent from the moment they are born. Remind them that they are in charge of their own bodies

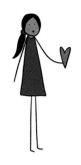

'Kindness was always at the core of girl power'

Victoria Beckham OBE,

Singer, fashion designer and television personality

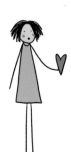

RAIN, RAIN, GO AWAY

'Now more than ever in our lifetimes we need to show kindness to each other, rather than focusing on the things which divide us. I believe being kind and showing empathy is the first step towards overcoming the anger and frustration that seems to be all around right now.'

Sir Chris Hoy MBE,

Olympic champion track cyclist

Kindness is sharing our stories

'Some have bravely shared their stories; they have opened the door, knowing that when one person speaks truth, it gives license for all of us to do the same. We have learned that when people ask how any of us are doing, and when they really listen to the answer, with an open heart and mind, the load of grief often becomes lighter – for all of us. In being invited to share our pain, together we take the first steps toward healing.' [6]

The Duchess of Sussex

Kindness is anti-racist

'Through understanding our shared humanity, let's make kindness a part of everything we do. Be mindful of your actions and dare to be different. Stand up for what is right, even when it is difficult to do so.'

June Sarpong OBE,

Diversity expert and author

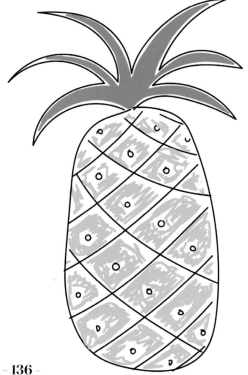

BE KIND:

How to be anti-racist:

- Hold your friends and family accountable: challenge yourself to engage in conversations with those close to you when they make problematic comments

- Come to terms with your own privilege. Reading up on this is a good place to start

- Diversify your knowledge and check your information bias: subscribe to newsletters focused on racial equality and amend your news outlets to include different viewpoints and ideologies

- Do not use comments that are based on stereotypical assumptions

- Educate yourself about the history of racism

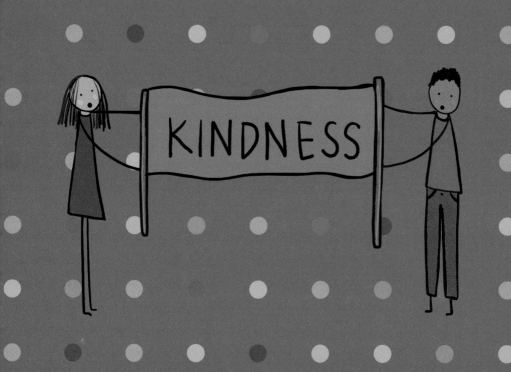

'I feel like what the world needs is a revolution of kindness, of inner kindness and compassion towards each other and the planet as opposed to violent and bloody revolution. I don't think that revolution can come from any other source but within us. I don't think there are answers in politics or religion. I think it has to come from the people themselves.'

Paul Weller,

Singer, songwriter and musician

Wear kind clothing

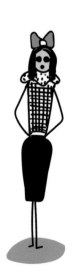

'Kindness will never go out of fashion'

Caroline Rush CBE,

CEO of the British Fashion Council

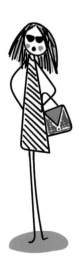

BE KIND:

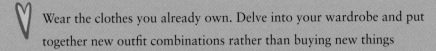

♡ Wear the clothes you already own. Delve into your wardrobe and put together new outfit combinations rather than buying new things

♡ Garment swap with friends and family – you both get something new!

♡ Invest in clothes that will see you through more than one season

♡ Shop in charity or vintage shops

♡ Do your best to shop with brands who pay their workers a fair living wage, in environments where they feel safe

♡ Rent clothes for special occasions

♡ Find out where brands source their materials and how sustainable their production process is

♡ Save up for quality pieces. Buy less fast fashion

♡

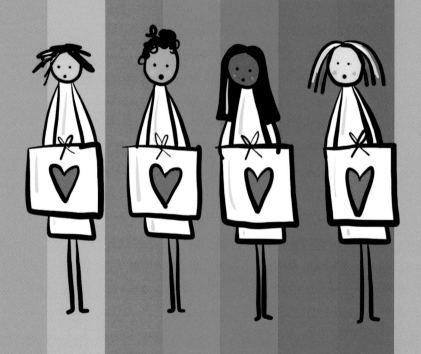

'We sometimes think the world's problems are so big that we can do little to help. On our own, we cannot end wars or wipe out injustice, but the cumulative impact of thousands of small acts of goodness can be bigger than we imagine.'[7]

Queen Elizabeth II

Show kindness to animals

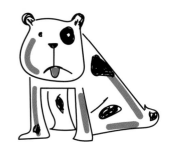

Spending time with pets reduces stress and cholesterol as well as feelings of anxiety and depression. Show the same kindness to animals as you would to humans.

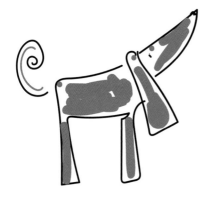

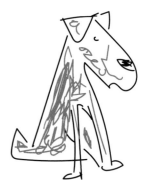

BE KIND:

- Shop cruelty-free by ensuring that your products aren't tested on animals
- Sponsor an animal living in a shelter
- Take a trip to a beach and litter-pick to protect ocean wildlife
- Respect wild animals and leave them and their habitat be
- Avoid feeding animals you see when out as this could damage their health
- Set up a bird box in your garden or a shelter for hedgehogs
- If you eat meat, make sure that it is organic, ethical and from local farms
- Go out of your way to cuddle all the animals in your life – it will feel good for both of you!
- Consider getting your next pet from an animal rescue organisation

'A single act of kindness throws out roots in all directions, and the roots spring up and make new trees.' [8]

Amelia Earhart,

Aviation pioneer and author

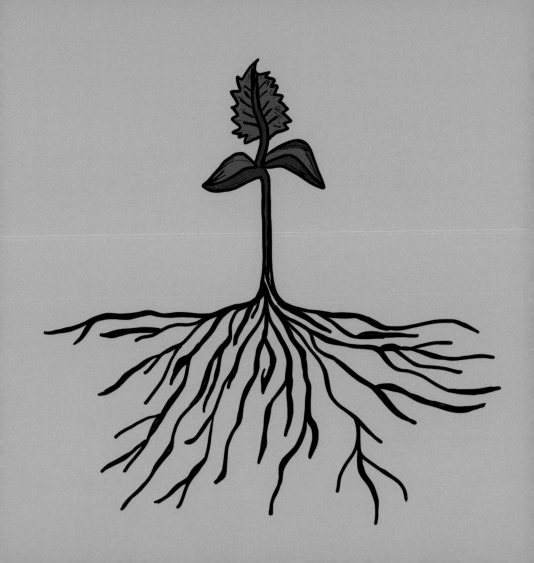

Eco-chic entertaining

'Having a kinder, more patient and tolerant approach to life is a crucial healing tool. Particularly in challenging times. As an eco event organiser and founder of a sustainable business, I believe that the key to a more sustainable future has to be a circular approach. We need to be kinder to the planet and the people in it all at once.'

Yasmin Mills,

Eco events organiser and founder of Ecofêtes sustainable homeware

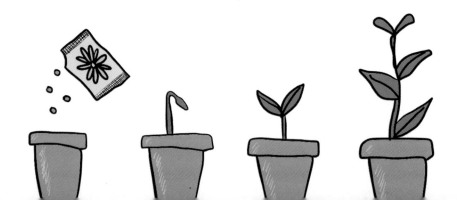

BE KIND:

Here are Yasmin's tips for sustainable, chic eco-entertaining:

1 Choose your menu before you go shopping. Whether you are having a family dinner party or canapés and cocktails at home, make a list of exactly what you want to serve and to how many guests. To avoid unnecessary food waste, it's better to shop with a pre-planned list than a hungry tummy.

2 Avoid throwaway paper napkins or any plastic tableware that causes unnecessary waste. Whether vintage or new, invest in fabric table linen and beautiful glassware that can be reused for years.

3 Ensure your floral décor is multi-use. Rather than using flowers that die and get thrown away, decorate your space or dinner table with little potted plants that you will love and keep in your home long after the party is over.

4 Buy less, choose well, make it last. Whether it's a new party frock or tableware, buy well-made items that you will cherish and enjoy for years. Take time to find out not only how the new things you buy are made, but how the people making them are treated. A little online research and looking into a brand's sustainability statement on their website can usually tell you what you need to know.

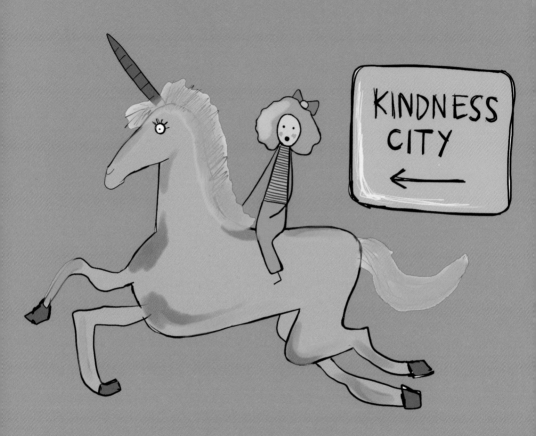

KINDNESS CREATES
THRIVING COMMUNITIES

Creating a space filled with kindness and positivity can help contribute to our sense of community. And that sense of belonging, studies have shown, can be a key contributor to living a longer, happier life.

'Kindness has many faces – compassion, forgiveness, gentleness, responsibility, friendship, inclusion, awareness and acceptance; however, kindness only becomes a life changing power when we act upon it.'

Jo Malone CBE,
Perfumer and founder of Jo Malone London

Kindness can save lives

'Kindness seems to be such an undervalued trait, but it is the thing that can make or break you in life. Kindness has a particular poignancy to me because – as a victim of coercive abuse – I felt I lived in a world without it for almost ten years throughout my marriage. I was isolated from friends and family and every day I would be told awful things about myself, by the man who was supposed to love me. "You look fat, you look old, you look ugly, everyone thinks you're stupid. Everyone hates you." Those words, those constant unkind, abusive words damaged me more than any kick or punch and took so much longer to heal from.

I am now a patron of Women's Aid and doing everything I can to raise awareness about domestic abuse. Like so many other victims, I am still recovering. I have my family and friends around me once more and I appreciate more than ever the power of kindness that has been shown to me by them, by all of those involved in Women's Aid and even strangers who write to me thanking me for bringing this subject to light with my book, *Brutally Honest*. Kindness costs nothing but it can be the most precious gift.' [9]

Melanie B,

Singer, television personality and actress

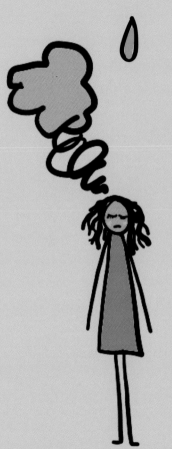

'Kindness officially means the quality of being friendly, generous and considerate. Other words associated with kindness include affection, gentleness, warmth, concern and care. Kindness is also in the compassion and empathy camp. It's a good gang to be part of. If you are yet to jump on board the kindness bus, you might want to hop on at the next stop. Being kind will instantly make you feel better about yourself and your place in the world. Like a drug, except legal and with only positive side effects. And with that in mind, what if kindness becomes addictive? How cool would that be? Or what if it already has but the people who run the news don't want us to know because it will be the end of all bad news forever and they might be out of a job. Don't delay, be kind today.'

Chris Evans,

Radio DJ

The Cranes Are Back

By **Paul Weller**

The cranes are back
Say the cranes are back
Go tell your momma
Tell her spread the news

Tell 'em that the cranes are back
There ain't no chains on my back
There ain't no chains on my back
There's only joy that freedom brings
Tell 'em that the cranes are back

Been a long time making a show
And all this winter going so slow
Cause a kind reaction so
We could feel the love once more

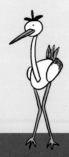

They're all flying back

They're all flying back

Come see the sky

Hear the people cry

Get running, say the cranes are back

Cranes are back

Been a long time making a show

And all this winter going so slow

Form a kind revolution so

From that hope and a new
  world born

Pick ourselves up off the floor

Try to heal the land once more

Cause a kind reaction so

There would be some hope in
  the world

It's been a long time making a show

Crops and water plentiful

Babies washed up on the shore

War and hatred more and more

Start a kind revolution so...

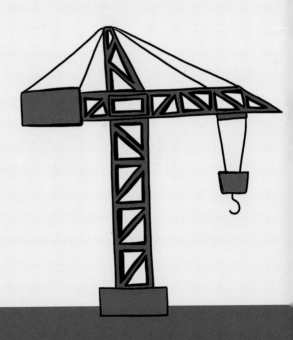

Finally, believe that you alone are 'enough' and keep your cup full to the brim with kindness in every interaction you have, and life will be kind to you in return. That's when the magic happens.

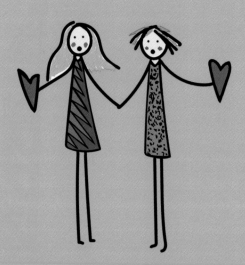

Rosie's acknowledgements

A million thanks to my talented collaborator Jakki Jones – this has been a dream partnership and I am so lucky to count you as a friend.

A huge thank you to Kate Ansell for being so integral to the research and writing process. When I was feeling like there weren't enough hours in the day, you kindly stepped in to help and your excitement for it shone through.

To Lisa Milton at HQ Stories for believing in the great goodness of this book and agreeing to publish it. Jakki and I both want to thank our fabulous editors Kate Fox and Abigail Le Marquand-Brown and designer Steve Wells, for lovingly turning it into a work of art; plus, my agent Jenny Savill for the encouragement. Warm and fuzzy feelings all round!

Hugs and gratitude to all the personalities and experts who made time to consider kindness and write such beautiful, thoughtful words for this book.

To my parents, thank you for leading by example – your kindness has made me strong – and I will proudly carry on the legacy of 'kindness no matter what' left by my beloved grandma.

This book wouldn't have come to life without the encouragement of my husband, Callum. Thank you for the kindness you always show me and our family, and the support you give me to realise my passion projects.

And finally, to my sons Heath and Rex, watching you grow into empathetic young men is a privilege and I am so proud of your kind hearts. I love you.

Jakki's acknowledgements

I'd like to thank my Mum and Dad for giving me the gift of kindness. You taught my sisters (Linda and Sandra) and I to always be kind in life and for that I am so grateful. Love you so much.

This book is dedicated to my children; Riley, Marley, Misty and Colby, whom I love with all my heart, and who I hope will continue to spread kindness wherever they go, and finally for my husband Kelly – who is the kindest person I know.

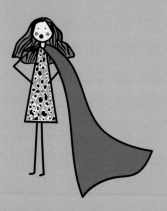

Notes and references

1   Malcolm X. A Declaration of Independence. 12 March 1964, New York City.

2   https://www.futurity.org/kindness-happiness-anxiety-2019962/, accessed 7 April 2021

3   The Duchess of Cambridge. Place2Be's 'Big Assembly'. 6 February 2017, Mitchell Brook Primary School, Brent.

4   His Holiness the 14th Dalai Lama of Tibet. Visit to Capitol Hill. 7 March 2014, Washington DC.

5   Desmond Tutu, *Hope and Suffering: Sermons and Speeches* (Wm. B. Eerdmans Publishing Company, 1984)

6   https://www.nytimes.com/2020/11/25/opinion/meghan-markle-miscarriage.html, accessed 7 April 2021

7   Her majesty the Queen. The Queen's Christmas Message. 25 December 2016, Buckingham Palace.

8   https://www.ameliaearhart.com/quotes/, accessed 7 April 2021

9   If you, or anyone you know has been affected by domestic abuse a good place to start is by referring them to https://www.womensaid.org.uk/ where there is an instant messaging service and an online forum. Or calling the freephone National Domestic Abuse Helpline 0808 2000 247